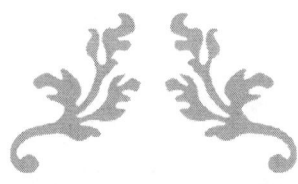

MAJOR SIX MARATHONS JOURNEY

Chicago Marathon

Table of Contents

Introduction

Running the Windy City – A Complete Guide to the Chicago Marathon

The marathon, an ancient distance of 26.2 miles, has captivated the world and continues to do so through events like the Abbott World Marathon Majors. This series of six elite races – in Berlin, Boston, Chicago, London, New York, and Tokyo – represents the pinnacle of marathon achievement, each city offering a unique backdrop for runners to test their physical limits and embrace the spirit of the marathon. Among these, the Chicago Marathon stands out not only for its place in the series but for its unique blend of history, culture, and sheer flat-out fast course. This book is a guide for anyone aiming to conquer the Chicago Marathon, whether you're a seasoned marathoner, a first-time runner, or simply interested in the legacy of one of the world's most storied races.

Chicago, known as the "Windy City," is home to nearly three million residents and a marathon that has long been famous for its fast, flat course. It's a city deeply rooted in cultural diversity, rich history, and a modern spirit that fuels innovation and progress. Runners from across the globe descend upon the city each October, ready to experience the sights, sounds, and excitement of racing through neighborhoods like Chinatown, Pilsen, and Old Town, each with its own identity and character. The Chicago Marathon has grown exponentially since its inception in 1977, when a relatively modest crowd of 4,200 runners toed the starting line. Now, nearly 50,000 participants line up each year, transforming the city into a living, breathing track dedicated to the marathon's grueling 26.2 miles.

The Prestige of the Abbott World Marathon Majors

The Abbott World Marathon Majors brings together six of the most famous marathons on the planet, where elite and amateur runners alike compete to earn points and ultimately claim the elusive Six-Star Finisher Medal. Within the series, the Chicago Marathon is known for its course speed and is one of the few major races where multiple world records have been set. The Major Six are as much a cultural and athletic experience as they are a testament to endurance, and runners of all levels travel worldwide for the chance to complete each one. In 2006, when Chicago officially became part of the World Marathon Majors, it solidified its place among the world's best marathons, attracting top-tier talent and everyday runners alike to the Windy City.

A Marathon for Every Runner

The Chicago Marathon's course, known for being flat and fast, is particularly appealing for both seasoned athletes looking to set a personal best and first-time marathoners who are less intimidated by the lack of steep hills. Chicago's marathon is not only accessible due to its course but also welcoming in its atmosphere. The race is known for its diverse runners and spectators, and its course takes participants through 29 neighborhoods, each providing a distinct flavor of Chicago life. Whether you're there to achieve a PR or simply complete the distance, the Chicago Marathon has something to offer everyone. It's no wonder runners return to Chicago year after year to compete again, often bringing family and friends to witness or join in the festivities.

The Growth and Impact of the Chicago Marathon

Starting from its modest beginnings in 1977, the Chicago Marathon has grown into an internationally recognized event, one of the largest marathons in the world by participant size. The race's history is filled with fascinating moments: the blistering course records, unforgettable weather conditions, and stories of perseverance from runners of all backgrounds. From its early days, the marathon aimed to be inclusive, encouraging people from all walks of life to run, walk, or wheel their way through the city. The growth of the marathon has helped the city itself, bringing significant tourism revenue and community pride.

Chicago's Unique Course and Character

A huge part of what makes Chicago's marathon unique is the course itself. The race begins and ends in Grant Park, Chicago's iconic lakefront gathering place, where runners enjoy stunning views of Lake Michigan and the towering skyscrapers that define the Chicago skyline. The course is designed to showcase the city's unique character, leading runners past famous landmarks and lively neighborhoods, each section contributing its own personality to the race. The neighborhoods aren't just passive parts of the course; the people who live there actively support runners by providing entertainment, cheers, and encouragement. From the classic architecture of the Loop to the colorful, cultural streets of Pilsen and Little Italy, the course offers a visual tour of Chicago's diversity and history.

The unpredictability of the October weather in Chicago also adds to the excitement. The city is known for its varied weather, and race day can bring anything from chilly winds and rain to unseasonably warm temperatures. This factor can affect race strategies and timing, but it also makes the experience memorable. For runners who enjoy a challenge, Chicago's marathon offers both the allure of a personal best and the thrill of dealing with whatever nature decides to bring that day.

Why Run the Chicago Marathon?
For many runners, the draw of the Chicago Marathon lies in the thrill of running a world-class event with unmatched energy and community support. It's an experience that goes beyond simply running 26.2 miles; it's about being part of a shared journey with tens of thousands of fellow runners and the people of Chicago. The marathon is an opportunity to test one's limits, meet new people, and revel in the joy of shared accomplishment. Whether you're running for a personal goal, to raise funds for a cause, or simply to be part of something bigger than yourself, the Chicago Marathon offers a chance to achieve something meaningful.

Running the Chicago Marathon is a personal journey, yet it is one shared by an entire city, a worldwide community, and the history that has made the event what it is today. For anyone who has ever wanted to run a marathon, especially a major one, Chicago is a perfect choice. It's inclusive, well-organized, and supported by enthusiastic crowds, making it one of the most accessible and welcoming marathons in the world.

What to Expect in This Book

This book will guide you through the entire process of preparing for, experiencing, and recovering from the Chicago Marathon. Each chapter is designed to provide you with insights, advice, and inspiration tailored to runners of all levels. You'll learn about the course layout, the history of the race, training tips, and advice for handling the unique challenges that come with running in the Windy City. You'll also find chapters dedicated to first-time marathoners and experienced runners who are looking to improve their performance.

Our goal is to equip you with all the tools and knowledge you need to make the most of your Chicago Marathon experience. From training plans to race-day strategies, this book covers it all, with advice from experienced runners and coaches who know the course inside and out. Whether you're aiming for a specific time goal, running to finish, or simply soaking in the experience, you'll find guidance that will help you cross that finish line with confidence.

So lace up your running shoes, set your sights on Grant Park, and get ready to take on the

Chicago Marathon. The Windy City awaits, ready to cheer you on every step of the way.

Chapter 1: History of the Chicago Marathon

The Chicago Marathon is one of the world's six major marathons, alongside Boston, New York, London, Berlin, and Tokyo. Known for its flat, fast course and the fervor of its spectators, the Chicago Marathon has evolved over nearly half a century into one of the most popular races worldwide, drawing participants from across the globe. But to understand its significance today, it's essential to delve into the history and development that transformed a local race into an internationally celebrated event. This chapter explores the marathon's origins, its struggles and triumphs, and the ways it has mirrored Chicago's growth, resilience, and diversity over the decades.

The Humble Beginnings

The roots of the Chicago Marathon trace back to the 1970s, a decade marked by a surge of interest in long-distance running across the United States. This "running boom" was partly due to American Frank Shorter's victory in the 1972 Olympic marathon, which inspired countless people to take up the sport. In Chicago, the popularity of running began to grow, especially as citywide interest in sports and fitness took hold.

Chicago's first marathon race, however, actually predates the current iteration of the Chicago Marathon by several years. The original marathon, held in 1905, was an unofficial race organized by the Illinois Athletic Club and took place along a 24.8-mile course. This event drew an enthusiastic crowd and was considered a great success, but it did not become an annual event. For decades, the city lacked an official marathon, although smaller races and running events became common. It wasn't until 1977 that the first official "modern" Chicago Marathon took place, marking the beginning of an era.

1977: The Inaugural "Mayor Daley Marathon"

The marathon was reborn on September 25, 1977, under the official name "Mayor Daley Marathon," in honor of the late Richard J. Daley, who had served as Chicago's mayor for over two decades. The Chicago Marathon's creation was largely the result of efforts by Lee Flaherty, an advertising executive and runner, who believed that the city needed an event that could showcase its neighborhoods, bring people together, and promote health and fitness. Flaherty, alongside co-founder Wendell "Wendy" Miller and others, worked to raise sponsorships and funding to turn their vision into reality.

The first Mayor Daley Marathon had approximately 4,200 participants, a remarkable turnout for a new race. Registration cost just $5, and the race attracted runners from various backgrounds and fitness levels, a testament to the growing appeal of marathon running in the U.S. While the first race was chaotic, it was an immediate success and put Chicago on the map in the marathon world. This first race laid the groundwork for the transformation of Chicago into a major marathon destination.

Expanding the Vision: The Early Years of the Chicago Marathon

In its early years, the Chicago Marathon quickly grew in popularity. In 1978, the race was renamed the "Chicago Marathon," shedding its political association and focusing on becoming a premier race. By 1979, the number of runners had nearly doubled to 8,000. The marathon's growth reflected the rising interest in running, as people began to see marathons not just as competitions but as personal achievements and testaments to resilience.

The late 1970s and early 1980s also marked the beginning of sponsorships that would play a crucial role in the race's development. Beatrice Foods became the first major sponsor, providing essential financial support that allowed the race to expand, increase its prize pool, and attract elite international runners. The influx of elite runners helped raise the marathon's prestige, and by the early 1980s, it had become one of the fastest-growing marathons in the world.

Challenges and Changes in the 1980s

The Chicago Marathon faced its share of challenges during the 1980s, especially after Beatrice Foods withdrew its sponsorship in 1985. The loss of major financial backing led to several difficult years, with rumors circulating that the race might be discontinued. However, organizers managed to secure other sponsors, though on a smaller scale, allowing the race to continue.

One of the defining moments of this era was the 1984 race, which saw Steve Jones of the UK set a world record with a time of 2:08:05. This record reinforced Chicago's reputation as a "fast course" and attracted more elite runners interested in breaking records and setting personal bests. Steve Jones's achievement showed that the Chicago Marathon was not only a great race but a world-class event capable of hosting the sport's best athletes. This record became a cornerstone in Chicago's journey to becoming a marathon powerhouse.

The Boom of the 1990s: Sponsorship and Growth

In 1994, a crucial partnership was established with the LaSalle Bank, marking a new chapter of financial stability and growth. With its new name, the LaSalle Bank Chicago Marathon, and increased funding, the race was now positioned to expand further and solidify its place among the top marathons globally. The prize money increased, and the marathon began investing more in logistics, medical facilities, and participant amenities. This financial support also allowed for marketing efforts that attracted even more participants, both domestically and internationally.

The 1990s also saw a push for inclusivity within the Chicago Marathon. The organizers began emphasizing the importance of diversity and accessibility, encouraging runners from various backgrounds and skill levels to participate. Wheelchair racers and disabled athletes became an integral part of the race, marking Chicago as one of the most inclusive marathons in the world.

Chicago's flat and fast course became particularly attractive for elite athletes seeking record-breaking performances. Several course records and personal bests were set during this period, solidifying the Chicago Marathon's reputation as one of the fastest courses in the world. By the end of the 1990s, the marathon had achieved international acclaim, ranking among the top marathons in the world.

Entering the 21st Century: Becoming a World Marathon Major

The Chicago Marathon entered the 21st century with tremendous momentum. In 2006, it achieved the status of being one of the "World Marathon Majors" (WMM), joining the ranks of Boston, New York, Berlin, London, and Tokyo. This recognition brought an influx of international media attention and elite runners, enhancing the marathon's profile globally.

Achieving WMM status also increased the Chicago Marathon's appeal to a new generation of runners who wanted to complete the "big six" marathons. The honor of running in one of the WMM races added to the event's allure, making it a must-run race for marathon enthusiasts. The organization invested in technology, like real-time runner tracking and social media updates, to connect with participants and spectators, offering a more interactive experience.

Recent Years: The Modern-Day Chicago Marathon

The modern-day Chicago Marathon continues to grow, attracting a diverse group of runners and spectators. The Bank of America took over sponsorship in 2008, bringing additional resources and visibility to the race. The marathon now draws over 40,000 participants annually and is watched by approximately 1.7 million spectators along the course.

In recent years, the marathon has placed a strong emphasis on environmental sustainability and community involvement. The race organizers have introduced several green initiatives, such as recycling waste, reducing plastic usage, and encouraging runners to use public transportation. Additionally, the marathon collaborates with local organizations and charities, raising millions of dollars for various causes each year. This commitment to community and sustainability reflects the evolving values of the marathon and its participants.

Achievements and Milestones

The Chicago Marathon has been the site of several landmark performances over the years. In 2019, Brigid Kosgei of Kenya set the women's world record with a time of 2:14:04, breaking Paula Radcliffe's long-standing record. This achievement cemented Chicago's reputation as one of the fastest marathon courses in the world.

Throughout its history, the Chicago Marathon has also had its share of memorable finishes and emotional moments, from runners overcoming personal adversity to dramatic final sprints. Each year, the marathon brings together thousands of stories of resilience, determination, and the human spirit.

A Symbol of Chicago's Resilience and Spirit

Today, the Chicago Marathon stands as a symbol of the city's resilience, diversity, and community spirit. From its humble beginnings to its current status as one of the World Marathon Majors, the race reflects Chicago's journey as a city that has weathered challenges and emerged stronger. Each year, the marathon unites people from all over the world, connecting them through the shared challenge of running 26.2 miles. It has become more than just a race; it's a celebration of endurance, a showcase of Chicago's neighborhoods, and a testament to the city's commitment to excellence.

For both Chicagoans and visitors, the marathon is a cherished event that represents the best of the city. The race continues to grow, attracting new generations of runners who come to experience its legendary course, unparalleled support, and the welcoming spirit of Chicago. The marathon's history is a living story, one that evolves with each race and each runner who crosses the finish line.

Chapter 2: The Heart of Chicago - A Journey through the Marathon's Iconic Course

Running the Chicago Marathon is more than just a race; it's a unique tour of the city that connects runners to the heart and soul of Chicago. Over the years, the marathon has earned a reputation for its scenic course, flat terrain, and incredible support from Chicagoans who line the streets, cheering on every participant. Each neighborhood along the route offers its own cultural flavor, historical significance, and energy, giving runners an unforgettable experience as they pass through 26.2 miles of diverse Chicago streets. This chapter delves deep into the neighborhoods, landmarks, and sights that runners encounter, providing a mile-by-mile breakdown of what to expect and how to prepare.

The Start at Grant Park

Every year, tens of thousands of runners gather in Grant Park, excited and nervous as they await the start. Located on the edge of Lake Michigan, Grant Park is one of Chicago's iconic spaces, stretching over 300 acres with incredible views of the skyline. As dawn breaks, runners gather with the excitement in the air palpable. The park itself is steeped in Chicago history and serves as the perfect setting to begin this journey.

The early miles weave through downtown Chicago, where towering skyscrapers and historic architecture greet runners. These initial miles are full of cheers and encouragement from spectators who line the streets, many of them family and friends who came to support. The excitement of the crowd provides an incredible boost, helping runners shake off pre-race jitters. The feeling of being surrounded by so many people who share the same goal of conquering 26.2 miles is both humbling and invigorating.

Downtown Loop and the Financial District (Miles 1–4)

The first few miles take runners through Chicago's financial heart, the Loop, famous for its towering buildings and lively atmosphere. This section includes iconic buildings like the Willis Tower, formerly known as the Sears Tower, which stands as a testament to the city's architectural prowess. Running through the Loop is exhilarating, as the cityscape seems to soar around you, while spectators crowd the streets to cheer runners on.

The Financial District, rich in history, also boasts a fascinating landscape of modern-day skyscrapers juxtaposed with art deco and beaux-arts architecture. These early miles are fast-paced and lively, with the buzz of the city at full tilt. Runners can hear cheers echo off the tall buildings, amplifying the excitement. It's an area where runners need to pace themselves; the adrenaline can make it easy to start too fast, but it's essential to conserve energy for later miles.

The River North and Near North Side (Miles 5–8)

As runners head north, they enter the vibrant River North and Near North Side neighborhoods, famous for their art galleries, chic restaurants, and historic landmarks. This part of the course is known for its fantastic crowd support, with spectators eagerly lining the streets, ringing bells, and holding encouraging signs. The area's artistic vibe is reflected in murals, unique storefronts, and lively, colorful streets, keeping runners visually engaged.

The Near North Side also offers views of the Chicago River and the striking bridges that cross it. This scenic section can be an emotional part of the race, as the river's calm provides a brief mental escape from the rigors of running. Many runners find a sense of flow here, getting into their stride and connecting with the city around them.

Lincoln Park and the Zoo (Miles 9–12)

Lincoln Park, one of Chicago's largest green spaces, offers a beautiful contrast to the city's urban environment. Running through the park's winding paths, under the shade of towering trees, is a serene experience. The Lincoln Park Zoo, located within the park, is home to a variety of animals and is one of the oldest zoos in the country. Though the zoo isn't part of the race, knowing it's nearby adds a layer of charm to this section of the course.

This part of the race can feel like a mental breather. The cooler air under the trees, coupled with a slight decline in the noise level, allows runners to gather their thoughts and focus on the next segment. Lincoln Park is also a popular spot for local runners, and many residents come out to offer a more intimate form of encouragement, calling out individual names and providing water and snacks.

Old Town and Boystown (Miles 13–15)

As runners approach the halfway point, they enter Old Town and Boystown, neighborhoods known for their vibrant energy and colorful character. Boystown, in particular, is a highlight, celebrated for its inclusivity and support of the LGBTQ+ community. The spectators here are some of the most enthusiastic and creative, often dressing in costumes and dancing along the sidelines. Their cheers provide a second wind for many runners just when they need it most.

Old Town, with its historical architecture and well-preserved brownstones, gives runners a glimpse of old Chicago charm. This section of the course is lively and engaging, with both neighborhoods bringing a festive energy that reinvigorates runners as they pass through. Here, the crowd's energy is tangible, lifting spirits as runners head toward the back half of the course.

Heading West through Diverse Neighborhoods (Miles 16–20)

In these miles, the course moves westward, taking runners through neighborhoods like Little Italy, University Village, and Pilsen. Little Italy offers a taste of Chicago's Italian-American heritage, with Italian restaurants and a strong sense of community lining the route. The University Village, home to the University of Illinois at Chicago, brings a youthful, academic vibe to the race, with students cheering on runners from the sidelines.

Pilsen is one of the most memorable parts of the course. Known for its Hispanic heritage, Pilsen bursts with color, from its murals to the lively Mexican music that fills the streets. This is a culturally rich area where residents bring their unique energy to the marathon, making runners feel as though they are part of a joyous citywide festival. These miles can be challenging, but the energy and support from the community help push runners forward.

Chinatown and the Bridgeport Area (Miles 21–23)
By the time runners reach Chinatown, fatigue often sets in, but the neighborhood's vibrant atmosphere provides an incredible morale boost. The Chinese arches, red lanterns, and the aroma of delicious food in the air create an immersive experience. Chinatown's community rallies around the marathon, providing music, dance, and endless cheering.

Bridgeport, a working-class neighborhood with deep roots in Chicago's labor history, follows Chinatown. While not as flashy, Bridgeport's community members are steadfast supporters of the marathon, offering encouragement and often reminding runners of how close they are to the finish. This stretch of the race is challenging, and the crowd's support here is crucial for helping runners press on.

The Final Stretch: South Loop and Grant Park Finish Line (Miles 24–26.2)

The last few miles bring runners through the South Loop, an area of modern high-rises and bustling city life. By now, exhaustion has set in, and runners must dig deep to keep going. The cheers grow louder, with the crowd sensing the effort and offering words of encouragement. As runners approach Grant Park, adrenaline kicks in. The sight of the skyline and the sound of the crowd build the anticipation, reminding runners of how far they've come.

Crossing the finish line in Grant Park is an emotional experience. Some runners sprint, others slow down to take it all in, but every finisher is met with a roar of applause and the satisfaction of knowing they've completed the Chicago Marathon. The finish line isn't just the end of the race; it's the culmination of months, sometimes years, of preparation and effort. Runners receive their medals, a symbol of their achievement and a reminder of their journey through the heart of Chicago.

Chapter 3: Preparing for the Chicago Marathon

Preparing for the Chicago Marathon is a journey of dedication, resilience, and strategy. Whether you're a seasoned marathoner or tackling your first marathon, the Chicago Marathon presents a unique set of challenges and opportunities. As a World Marathon Major, it attracts runners from around the globe, each with their own personal goals, but all with the same 26.2-mile course ahead. This chapter dives into the essential steps for successful preparation, from understanding the course layout and ideal training regimens to managing nutrition, rest, and race-day strategies.

Understanding the Course and Weather Conditions

One of the key aspects of preparing for the Chicago Marathon is familiarizing yourself with the course itself. The Chicago Marathon course is renowned for its flat and fast terrain, winding through 29 diverse neighborhoods. Runners often find this an ideal layout for attempting personal records (PRs) and qualifying times for other major marathons. However, the course's reputation as a "fast course" shouldn't lead runners to underestimate it; certain unique aspects require attention for optimal performance.

- **The Route**: The marathon begins in Grant Park and continues through areas like the Loop, Lincoln Park, and Pilsen before returning to the starting point. Each section has its distinct characteristics; for example, the early miles through downtown have more twists and turns, which can slow runners if not anticipated. The second half of the course becomes straighter, with long stretches that require consistent pacing and focus.

- **Weather Considerations**: Early October in Chicago can bring anything from high humidity to a crisp autumn chill. Average temperatures range from 45 to 65 degrees Fahrenheit, but fluctuations are common. Preparing for variable weather conditions is essential. Training in a range of temperatures, from hot days to cooler mornings, will help runners adapt to possible conditions on race day. Chicago's famous "windy city" breezes can also factor into the experience, especially as runners turn into more open areas; adjusting pace or drafting behind other runners in windy sections can help conserve energy.

Building a Training Plan

Training for a marathon requires a structured, consistent approach. While general fitness levels, running experience, and previous races may dictate slight variations in training plans, most marathon programs span 16 to 20 weeks, focusing on three major components: base-building, peak mileage, and tapering.

1 **Base-Building**: The first phase of training focuses on building a solid running foundation. This period emphasizes increasing weekly mileage at a manageable pace, which helps to improve cardiovascular endurance and strengthen muscles and joints gradually. During this stage, incorporating a mix of shorter and longer runs, including tempo runs and hill workouts, can increase stamina and endurance.

2 **Peak Mileage**: Approximately 8 to 10 weeks before race day, runners enter the peak mileage phase. Here, the weekly mileage reaches its highest points, often totaling between 35 to 50 miles or more for amateur runners and significantly more for seasoned athletes. Long runs become more critical, typically extending to 18–22 miles, helping runners become accustomed to sustained effort over long periods. This phase is challenging and

requires careful management of rest and nutrition to avoid injury or burnout.

3 **Tapering**: In the final 2-3 weeks before race day, tapering allows the body to recover while maintaining fitness levels. During this period, runners gradually reduce mileage but maintain the intensity of shorter runs to avoid feeling sluggish. Tapering ensures that the body is well-rested and ready for peak performance on race day, reducing muscle fatigue and mental burnout.

Training for the Chicago Marathon also benefits from strategic cross-training, such as cycling, swimming, or strength training. These activities improve overall fitness, prevent overuse injuries, and add variety to the routine.

Nutrition and Hydration Strategies

Nutrition is a cornerstone of marathon preparation, as proper fueling and hydration have a direct impact on training performance, recovery, and race-day success.

1 **Daily Nutrition**: During training, the body requires a balance of macronutrients: carbohydrates for energy, proteins for muscle repair, and fats for sustained fuel. Runners often increase their daily caloric intake to meet the demands of increased

mileage, emphasizing nutrient-dense foods like whole grains, lean proteins, healthy fats, and plenty of fruits and vegetables.

2 **Carbohydrate Loading**: In the days leading up to the marathon, many runners practice "carb-loading," a dietary approach where the intake of carbohydrates is increased to maximize glycogen stores. This strategy ensures that muscles have a readily available source of energy during the marathon, helping to prevent "hitting the wall" when glycogen stores deplete. For Chicago's race day, runners should begin carb-loading about 2-3 days before, while continuing to maintain hydration.

3 **Race-Day Fueling**: Fueling during the race is essential, as most runners cannot complete a marathon without replenishing energy stores. Energy gels, chews, or drinks are common, as they provide quick-digesting carbohydrates to sustain energy levels. Practicing race-day nutrition during long training runs allows runners to test their tolerance to different fuel sources, which minimizes the risk of gastrointestinal discomfort on race day.

4 **Hydration**: Hydration is equally important and can be adjusted based on weather

and sweat rates. Chicago Marathon organizers provide water and electrolyte stations every mile, allowing runners to stay hydrated throughout the race. Understanding personal hydration needs is crucial, and incorporating electrolyte-rich beverages, especially in warm conditions, helps replace sodium lost through sweat.

Managing Rest, Recovery, and Injury Prevention

Training for a marathon demands a careful balance between pushing the body to improve endurance and allowing it to recover. Rest and recovery practices reduce the risk of injury and improve overall performance.

- **Rest Days**: Including one or two rest days each week helps the body repair and strengthens muscles and joints, preventing overtraining syndrome. Some runners may find value in incorporating "active recovery" days, such as gentle yoga or light stretching, which promote circulation without straining the body.

- **Sleep**: Adequate sleep is vital for muscle repair and mental resilience, especially during peak training. Aim for 7-9 hours of quality sleep each night, particularly before long runs, as sleep plays a critical role in recovery and mental focus.

- **Injury Prevention**: Common injuries for marathon runners include shin splints, plantar fasciitis, and IT band syndrome. Preventive measures like stretching, foam rolling, and targeted strength exercises reduce the risk of these injuries. Paying attention to early signs of discomfort and consulting a physical therapist when needed can prevent minor issues from escalating.

Mental Preparation: Developing a Marathon Mindset

Mental toughness is a crucial element of marathon training. Preparing for and running a marathon requires focus, resilience, and determination, qualities that become especially important when physical fatigue sets in during the final miles.

1 **Visualization Techniques**: Visualizing the course and imagining a successful race helps prepare the mind for race day. Some runners find value in picturing specific landmarks along the course and mentally rehearsing how they'll feel and respond to various challenges.

2 **Setting Milestones**: Breaking down the race into smaller segments, such as the first 10 miles, the halfway point, or the 20-mile marker, can make the distance seem less daunting. Many marathoners focus on these milestones, congratulating themselves on each segment completed and staying motivated to tackle the next one.

3 **Mantras and Positive Self-Talk**: Adopting a positive mantra, such as "strong and steady" or "one mile at a time," helps sustain mental strength. Positive self-talk encourages the runner through difficult moments, preventing negative thoughts from undermining their focus.

4 **Training for the "Wall"**: The infamous "wall" often hits around mile 20, where glycogen stores deplete, and fatigue intensifies. Training through mental and physical fatigue, particularly during long runs, helps prepare the mind to push through this critical point. Knowing that the wall is a temporary challenge allows runners to mentally brace for it and push beyond.

Final Preparations and Race Day Strategy

In the weeks leading up to the marathon, runners should take specific steps to ensure a successful race day experience.

- **Race Kit and Gear Check**: Familiarity with race-day gear is essential, as new items can cause discomfort or chafing. Many runners conduct a "dress rehearsal" during a long run to test the outfit, shoes, and any other equipment they'll use on race day. Chicago's weather can be unpredictable, so having gear for varying conditions, like rain or cold, is prudent.

- **Logistics**: The Chicago Marathon has a vast organization, with designated start waves, bag check options, and specific parking guidelines. Reviewing these logistics well in advance ensures a smooth race-day experience. Runners should arrive early to allow time for stretching, gear checks, and finding their designated corral.

- **Pacing Strategy**: Proper pacing is essential in a marathon. For many runners, maintaining an even pace throughout the race prevents burnout. Chicago's course, with its flat terrain, is ideal for even pacing, but it's easy to start too quickly in the excitement of the early miles. Practicing race pace during training helps reinforce this rhythm, increasing the likelihood of a successful finish.

Chapter 4: Race Day Experience

Race day for the Chicago Marathon is an unforgettable experience. The energy in the city is palpable, as tens of thousands of runners and hundreds of thousands of spectators prepare to come together for an event that transcends athletics. The race draws participants from all over the world, each with their own goals, motivations, and dreams of reaching that 26.2-mile finish line. The Chicago Marathon's atmosphere is vibrant, with each of the city's neighborhoods adding unique cultural flavor to the journey, and the massive crowd provides an electrifying backdrop for runners as they navigate their way through the heart of the Windy City.

This chapter dives into the details of race day, from pre-race preparations and the excitement at the starting line to the rhythm of the race itself and the elation of crossing the finish line. Understanding what to expect on race day can help alleviate pre-race nerves and ensure that each participant can truly enjoy the experience.

Pre-Race Preparations

The morning of the Chicago Marathon is exhilarating yet filled with nerves. Most participants wake up before dawn to make their way to Grant Park, where the race begins. Getting to the park early is critical, as it allows time for last-minute preparations, stretching, and warming up before heading to the start corral.

- **Logistics and Arrival**: Since roads around Grant Park and the Loop close early, many participants opt to stay in nearby hotels or use public transportation. The Chicago Transit Authority (CTA) offers convenient transit options, including buses and the "L" train, making it easy for runners to arrive at the race site without the hassle of finding parking. Arriving at least an hour before the start time allows enough time to check bags, find the assigned corral, and take in the energy of the pre-race atmosphere.

- **Bag Drop and Gear**: The Chicago Marathon offers a bag check option, so runners can bring essential items for after the race, such as warm clothes, snacks, and recovery items. Checking bags early is advised to avoid crowds and ensure there's enough time for warm-up activities.

- **Last-Minute Nutrition and Hydration**: Many runners bring a pre-race snack to maintain energy levels and sip on water or sports drinks to stay hydrated.

Common choices include bananas, energy bars, or bagels with peanut butter. The goal is to eat something easily digestible about an hour before the race, giving the body time to process the food without causing discomfort.

- **Mental Preparation and Warm-Up**: Taking a few minutes for mental preparation can set a positive tone for the race. Visualization techniques—imagining oneself running strong and finishing with energy—can be powerful for mental focus. A light warm-up, such as jogging in place or dynamic stretches, helps loosen muscles and prepares the body for the effort ahead.

The Starting Line Excitement

The starting line of the Chicago Marathon is a spectacle in itself. With over 40,000 runners gathered in their respective corrals, the energy is electric. The crowd ranges from elite athletes vying for records to first-time marathoners and charity runners who have trained for months to reach this moment. The hum of excitement and anticipation fills the air, and it's common for nerves to mix with excitement in those last few moments before the race begins.

4 **Wave Starts and Corrals**: To manage the massive number of participants, the Chicago Marathon uses a wave start, with runners grouped into corrals based on their projected finish times. This approach not only alleviates congestion but also ensures that each runner can start at a comfortable pace. The start itself is staggered by about 10 to 15 minutes between waves, giving runners plenty of space on the course.

5 **The National Anthem and Countdown**: The marathon traditionally begins with the singing of the national anthem, followed by a countdown. As the race kicks off, each wave is cheered on by race officials and thousands of spectators, setting an inspiring tone for the miles ahead. For many runners, this is a surreal moment— a culmination of months of training and an official entry into one of the most respected marathons in the world.

6 **The First Mile**: The opening mile takes runners through the downtown streets of Chicago, with skyscrapers towering above and crowds lining both sides of the route. This section is particularly thrilling but can also be challenging, as the adrenaline rush can lead to a faster pace than intended. The key is to stay

mindful of pacing, as it's easy to get swept up in the excitement and start too fast, which can lead to burnout later.

The Rhythm of the Race

Once the initial excitement settles, runners find their rhythm. The Chicago Marathon course offers scenic views, cultural highlights, and crowd support that make it an enjoyable route. The flat terrain is advantageous for maintaining a steady pace, though pacing discipline remains essential to avoid energy depletion in the later miles.

5 **Scenic and Cultural Highlights·** The Chicago Marathon passes through 29 neighborhoods, each offering its own vibe. Runners move from the modern skyscrapers of the Loop to the historic architecture of Old Town, the tree-lined streets of Lincoln Park, and the colorful murals in Pilsen. Each neighborhood adds a unique flavor, with diverse spectators cheering on the runners with signs, costumes, and live music.

6 **Crowd Support and Cheering Sections**: One of the standout features of the Chicago Marathon is the incredible crowd support. Fans line almost every mile of the route, cheering on runners

with encouraging words, high-fives, and homemade signs. The enthusiasm is contagious and provides a psychological boost that helps runners push through challenging sections. The dedicated cheering sections, such as Boystown, Chinatown, and Pilsen, are known for their spirited support, adding to the excitement and motivation.

7 **Pacing and Energy Management**: Pacing is critical in a marathon, and the flat Chicago course makes it tempting to push the pace early on. However, experienced runners know the importance of conserving energy. Many follow a strategy of even or negative splits, where the first half of the race is run slightly slower than the second half. Fueling stations are located every 1-2 miles, offering water, sports drinks, and sometimes gels, allowing runners to hydrate and replenish energy at regular intervals.

The Challenges of the Final Miles

The last miles of the marathon are both physically and mentally demanding. This is the point where many runners encounter "the wall"—the point of extreme fatigue when the body's glycogen stores are nearly depleted. The

Chicago Marathon's flat course may not have physical hills, but the mental "hills" in these final miles can feel just as challenging.

- **The 20-Mile Marker**: Reaching mile 20 is a major milestone in any marathon. This is often where the body and mind begin to feel the strain of the distance, and self-doubt can creep in. The Chicago Marathon's final stretch requires mental toughness and determination. Runners often rely on mantras, personal motivations, or the encouragement of the crowd to stay focused during this segment.

- **Mind Over Matter**: For many, the last few miles are more mental than physical. Developing a positive mindset and reminding oneself of the accomplishment of finishing is essential. Visualizing crossing the finish line or recalling why one signed up for the race in the first place can be helpful motivators during these challenging miles. Crowd support is particularly impactful in this section, as cheers from spectators become even more meaningful as fatigue sets in.

- **Fuel and Hydration in the Final Stretch**: Proper fueling and hydration during earlier parts of the race help prevent severe energy dips, but runners may still need a final boost in the last miles. Small sips of sports drinks or a last energy gel can provide a lift, enabling runners to push through to the end.

Crossing the Finish Line

The Chicago Marathon finish line is located back at Grant Park, where the race began. Approaching the finish, runners experience a mix of emotions—relief, pride, and often, disbelief that they've conquered the 26.2 miles. Crossing the finish line is a momentous occasion, with volunteers, fellow runners, and loved ones cheering participants on as they complete the marathon.

5 **The Final Stretch**: The course takes runners along Michigan Avenue before the final turn onto Roosevelt Road, where a small incline leads to the last stretch. This final hill, though modest, can feel challenging after 26 miles, but the roar of the crowd helps push runners over the top and down to the finish line.

6 **Crossing the Finish Line**: Reaching the finish line is an overwhelming experience. Many runners raise their arms in victory, while others are overcome with emotion. The feeling of accomplishment, combined with the

physical relief of stopping, creates a powerful moment that's unique to marathon finishers.

7 **Post-Race Amenities and Recovery**: Once across the finish line, runners receive their finisher medals, a source of pride and a memento of the achievement. The marathon organizers provide water, sports drinks, and snacks to aid in recovery. Medical tents are available for those in need of immediate assistance, while post-race stretching and massage areas help runners ease their muscles.

8 **Celebration and Reflection**: Completing the Chicago Marathon is a monumental achievement, and many runners take time to celebrate with friends, family, or fellow participants. For some, the race is a personal best, while for others, it's a first-time finish. Reflecting on the journey, the challenges overcome, and the sights experienced on the course creates memories that last a lifetime.

Embracing the Marathon Spirit

The Chicago Marathon is as much a celebration as it is a race. The spectators, volunteers, and energy throughout the course bring a sense of unity and excitement. From the cheers in

Boystown to the energy of Chinatown, each neighborhood adds to the experience. Runners are encouraged to embrace the journey, taking in the cheers and sharing high-fives with the crowd.

Completing the Chicago Marathon is not just about crossing the finish line; it's the culmination of months of preparation, discipline, and endurance. The lessons learned in training and the race itself contribute to personal growth, resilience, and confidence. Preparing for the Chicago Marathon means investing in the physical, mental, and logistical aspects of the race, culminating in an experience that becomes part of a runner's lifelong memory. With proper preparation and dedication, each runner can enjoy the remarkable achievement of finishing one of the world's greatest races.

Chapter 5: Post-Race Recovery and Celebration

Completing the Chicago Marathon is an exhilarating achievement, one that fills runners with an immense sense of pride and accomplishment. However, crossing the finish line marks not only the end of the race but also the beginning of the critical post-race recovery period. Effective recovery is essential to help the body heal, prevent injuries, and prepare for future races or athletic goals. This chapter provides a comprehensive guide to post-race recovery and celebration, exploring the necessary steps to maximize healing, prolong the sense of accomplishment, and commemorate the unforgettable experience.

After dedicating months to training and enduring the 26.2 miles of the race, it's easy for runners to overlook the importance of recovery. Marathon recovery involves more than just resting; it includes nutrition, physical therapy, mental rejuvenation, and sharing the journey with loved ones and the running community. Here's how to approach each stage of post-race recovery and make the most of the celebrations.

1. Immediate Post-Race Care and Rehydration

As runners cross the finish line, the initial sense of relief is coupled with physical exhaustion. The body's energy reserves are severely depleted, and rehydrating and refueling are top priorities. During the race, the body expends immense energy, depletes glycogen stores, and loses fluids through sweat, so it's essential to replenish these resources right away.

- **Hydrate with Electrolytes**: After hours of exertion, the body is often low on electrolytes and fluids. Consuming water and electrolyte-rich drinks like sports beverages helps restore hydration levels and balances essential minerals like sodium, potassium, and magnesium. This process aids in preventing cramps and muscle fatigue.

- **Consume Simple Carbohydrates**: To restore glycogen levels, runners are encouraged to consume easily digestible carbohydrates within 30-60 minutes of finishing. Bananas, energy bars, and fruits are popular options provided in the post-race area to help initiate the recovery process.

- **Body Temperature Regulation**: After crossing the finish line, body temperature often drops rapidly, especially in cooler weather. Marathon organizers usually provide foil blankets to keep runners warm and prevent chills, which can help mitigate the risk of hypothermia.

2. Cool-Down and Stretching Routine

Following a marathon, the muscles are fatigued and susceptible to stiffness and soreness. Performing a gentle cool-down and stretching routine can alleviate some of the immediate discomfort and improve flexibility in the hours following the race.

7 **Light Walking**: While it might feel tempting to sit down immediately after finishing, walking for a few minutes helps maintain blood circulation and gradually brings the heart rate down. Light walking also helps in releasing lactic acid, a byproduct of muscle activity that contributes to soreness.

8 **Static Stretching**: Engaging in gentle static stretching can help improve blood flow to muscles and reduce post-race stiffness. Focus on the calves, hamstrings, quadriceps, and hip flexors, as these muscles bear most of the load during a marathon. Hold each stretch for about 20-30 seconds and avoid overstretching, as muscles are particularly vulnerable after prolonged strain.

9 **Foam Rolling**: Foam rolling the legs, back, and shoulders can reduce tension and relieve tight muscles. Foam rolling is best done a few hours after the race or the following day when the muscles have had some time to rest.

3. Refueling with Nutrient-Rich Foods

Proper nutrition is essential for muscle repair and overall recovery after a marathon. During the race, the body uses carbohydrates as a primary energy source, but protein, fats, vitamins, and minerals are also essential for restoring balance and healing damaged tissues.

8 **Carbohydrates for Glycogen Replenishment**: The body's glycogen stores are depleted after a marathon, so eating carbohydrate-rich foods like pasta, rice, bread, or oatmeal in the first meal post-race is vital. Consuming these within a few hours of finishing the marathon helps expedite muscle recovery.

9 **Protein for Muscle Repair**: Protein is crucial for repairing muscle fibers that may have been damaged during the run. Foods like chicken, eggs, beans, tofu, or a protein shake can provide the necessary protein for recovery. Aiming for a 3:1 ratio of carbohydrates to protein in the post-race

meal is a well-known formula for promoting muscle repair and energy replenishment.

10   **Antioxidant-Rich Foods**: Foods high in antioxidants, like berries, spinach, nuts, and dark chocolate, help combat the oxidative stress and inflammation that can occur after intense physical exertion. Including these in the post-race diet can speed up the body's healing process.

11   **Healthy Fats**: Incorporating healthy fats, such as those found in avocados, nuts, and olive oil, aids in reducing inflammation and provides a source of long-term energy that complements muscle recovery.

4. Rest and Recuperation

The body undergoes significant stress during a marathon, and giving it adequate time to rest is crucial for full recovery. Runners should prioritize sleep and avoid intense physical activity in the days following the race.

• **Quality Sleep**: Sleep is one of the most effective ways to promote recovery. During deep sleep, the body repairs muscle tissue and restores energy levels. Getting at least eight hours of sleep per night in the days following the marathon is recommended.

- **Active Rest**: While complete rest is essential, incorporating light activities like walking, gentle cycling, or swimming can improve blood circulation, which helps reduce muscle stiffness and aids in recovery. This is often referred to as "active recovery" and is most beneficial starting two to three days after the marathon.

- **Avoid Running**: It's generally advised to take a break from running for at least a week after a marathon. This allows muscles, joints, and connective tissues to fully heal and reduces the risk of overuse injuries.

5. Post-Race Emotional Recovery and Reflection

Marathons require mental resilience, and the post-race period can involve a mix of emotions—joy, relief, pride, and sometimes even a sense of emptiness now that the goal has been achieved. Taking time for reflection can help runners process these emotions and celebrate their accomplishment.

9 **Reflect on the Journey**: Writing down thoughts and feelings about the race experience, including the challenges and moments of triumph, can be therapeutic. Reflecting on the journey from training to race day helps create a sense of closure and appreciation for the dedication that went into achieving the goal.

10 **Celebrate the Achievement**: Whether it's through a quiet reflection or a celebration with family and friends, acknowledging the achievement is an important part of post-race recovery. Many runners choose to celebrate by going out for a meal or sharing their experience on social media, connecting with others who understand the significance of the accomplishment.

11 **Set New Goals**: Once recovered, many runners begin thinking about future goals. Setting new fitness or life goals provides a renewed sense of purpose and keeps motivation high. Whether it's another marathon, a shorter race, or a different fitness endeavor, establishing a new target can inspire ongoing personal growth.

6. Post-Race Physical Therapy and Injury Prevention

Marathons are taxing on the body, and even those who finish injury-free may still benefit from a post-race evaluation with a physical therapist. Addressing any potential issues early on can prevent long-term injuries.

- **Visit a Physical Therapist**: A physical therapist can identify any areas of concern, such as muscle imbalances, joint stress, or overuse injuries, and recommend specific exercises to strengthen weak areas. Physical therapy is especially beneficial for addressing potential injuries or soreness that may not be immediately noticeable.

- **Incorporate Recovery Exercises**: Depending on the runner's condition, physical therapists may suggest exercises like hip-strengthening movements, core workouts, or balance training. These exercises help prevent future injuries and improve overall running mechanics.

- **Massage Therapy**: Sports massages can alleviate soreness, release muscle tension, and reduce inflammation. Scheduling a massage within a few days of the marathon can enhance recovery and provide physical and mental relaxation.

7. Staying Connected with the Running Community

The Chicago Marathon fosters a sense of camaraderie among participants. Staying connected with the running community after race day can provide support and motivation as runners navigate their recovery journey.

- **Social Media and Online Forums**: Sharing experiences, race photos, and personal reflections on social media allows runners to celebrate together, even if they live far apart. Many find motivation and inspiration in the stories of others who share the same passion for running.

- **Join Running Clubs or Groups**: Connecting with local running clubs or groups can help maintain the sense of community that often forms during marathon training. Many clubs offer group runs, training programs, and events that keep runners motivated and engaged.

8. Honoring the Chicago Marathon Experience

The Chicago Marathon experience is a memorable milestone for all who participate. Many runners find ways to honor the race and commemorate the hard work they put into training and race day.

- **Display Medals and Race Memorabilia**: Displaying the race medal, bib, and other memorabilia is a popular way to celebrate the accomplishment. Shadow boxes, medal racks, and framed photos serve as reminders of the journey and the effort it took to achieve the marathon goal.

- **Document the Experience**: Writing a blog post, creating a scrapbook, or making a video documenting the race day experience allows runners to capture the memory in a creative and lasting way. Sharing the experience can also inspire others to take on the marathon challenge.

9. The Importance of Restorative Activities

In the weeks following the marathon, focusing on activities that support physical and mental recovery can be beneficial.

- **Yoga and Stretching**: Incorporating yoga or dedicated stretching sessions can improve flexibility, release tight muscles, and aid in relaxation. Yoga poses that target the legs, hips, and back are particularly beneficial for marathon recovery.

- **Mindfulness and Meditation**: The mental demands of marathon training and race day can lead to fatigue and stress. Practicing mindfulness or meditation helps runners decompress and mentally process the accomplishment.

Chapter 6: Chicago Marathon for First-Timers

Taking on the Chicago Marathon for the first time is an experience filled with excitement, nerves, and the unknown. As a first-timer, there are countless things to consider, from understanding the course to knowing what to expect on race day. This chapter provides a comprehensive guide tailored specifically for those who are new to this race, covering every aspect from pre-race preparation to post-race celebrations, offering advice on how to make the most of this unique opportunity.

1. Understanding the Course and Environment

One of the Chicago Marathon's biggest draws is its flat and fast course, which winds through the heart of the city, showcasing iconic neighborhoods and landmarks. However, running through a bustling metropolitan area like Chicago also presents unique challenges. The weather, for instance, can vary wildly in October. Some years have seen unseasonably hot conditions, while others have welcomed runners with cooler, ideal temperatures. The winds off Lake Michigan can also affect the race; it's helpful to be prepared for changing weather and unpredictable elements.

The course itself takes runners through a mixture of urban landscapes, from skyscraper-lined streets to tree-lined avenues, creating a sense of energy that's hard to match. For a first-timer, understanding these variables and how they might impact their performance is key. Study the course map in advance and familiarize yourself with major points along the way. Know where the aid stations are located and mentally divide the race into sections, as this will make the distance feel more manageable.

2. Training Plan for First-Timers

Preparing for a marathon is a serious commitment, and first-time marathoners should allow several months to train. Many beginner training plans last about 16-20 weeks, with a gradual increase in mileage to build endurance safely. Given Chicago's flat terrain, you can focus on maintaining a steady pace rather than navigating hills. However, incorporating some speedwork and strength training will be valuable in building resilience, especially if you are aiming to hit a certain time goal.

Consistency is key, so ensure that your schedule includes long runs, which typically occur once a week. These runs not only help condition your body to handle the distance but also help you mentally adjust to spending hours on your feet. In the weeks leading up to the race, follow a "tapering" period, where you gradually decrease mileage to allow your body to recover and reach peak performance on race day.

First-timers may also consider joining a running club or finding a training group for support. Many groups in Chicago specifically cater to marathon runners and can offer a structured training plan with guidance from experienced runners and coaches. Additionally, talking to seasoned marathoners can provide valuable insight into what to expect on race day, from the starting line experience to navigating post-race recovery.

3. Choosing the Right Gear

Ensuring you have the right gear is essential. The Chicago Marathon has diverse weather conditions, so choose breathable, moisture-wicking clothing and layer as needed. For beginners, testing your gear during training is important. Marathon day is not the time to try out a new pair of shoes, shorts, or nutrition strategy, as doing so could lead to blisters or discomfort that could hinder your experience. Opt for running shoes that provide comfort and support for long distances, and ensure they are properly broken in.

Chicago's spectators are famously supportive, and the atmosphere can be highly motivating.

However, this means you'll encounter noise, music, and cheering at various points along the course. Consider whether headphones will enhance your experience or if you'd rather immerse yourself fully in the environment.

4. Setting Realistic Goals

Setting achievable goals is crucial for first-timers. For some, simply finishing the marathon is an accomplishment, while others may have a specific time in mind. Whatever your goal, ensure it's realistic based on your training progress. Keep in mind that it's common for first-time marathoners to underestimate the mental and physical demands of running 26.2 miles. A helpful approach for beginners is to set a primary goal (e.g., finishing the race), a secondary goal (e.g., hitting a certain time), and an aspirational goal (e.g., setting a personal record).

While the race is known for its flat course and personal-best potential, it's best to avoid putting too much pressure on yourself. Approach the race with a mindset of celebration and achievement, rather than stress and rigid expectations.

5. Managing Pre-Race Jitters

Nervousness is natural, especially in the days leading up to your first marathon. To keep these nerves in check, stick to familiar routines and focus on logistics. Pick up your race bib and packet at the Chicago Marathon expo a day or two before race day, allowing yourself time to explore the event without rushing. This expo is also a great opportunity to connect with other first-timers and experienced marathoners, pick up last-minute gear, and get inspired by the scale and excitement of the event.

Prepare a checklist for race day, including items like your bib, timing chip, shoes, and nutrition, so you can head to the starting line feeling calm and organized. Make sure to get adequate rest in the days leading up to the race and stay hydrated.

6. The Starting Line Experience

The starting line can feel overwhelming for first-time runners, as thousands of runners gather in Grant Park to await the beginning of the race. Arriving early is essential, as there will be security checkpoints, gear check-in, and time to get settled in your designated corral. Embrace the energy around you, but remember to pace yourself. Adrenaline will be high, but it's crucial not to start too fast, which could lead to burnout later.

Take advantage of this moment to soak in the excitement. Many first-time runners report feeling a blend of anticipation and joy as they wait for the starting horn. Engage in the camaraderie around you, and keep your mental focus on the journey ahead rather than getting swept up in the fast pace of other runners.

7. Tackling Race-Day Challenges

Every marathon presents its challenges, and Chicago is no exception. First-time runners often encounter "the wall" around miles 18-22, where both physical and mental fatigue set in. Prepare for this by staying consistent with your hydration and nutrition plan, consuming fluids and energy gels or snacks at regular intervals. Knowing that this tough moment is likely to come can make it easier to push through.

Mentally, breaking down the course into manageable segments can help. Focus on reaching the next aid station, mile marker, or neighborhood, rather than thinking about the entire remaining distance. Drawing energy from the spectators and landmarks can also be a powerful motivator. For instance, seeing family and friends in the crowd or reaching a known milestone like Chinatown can help reinvigorate your spirit and keep you moving.

8. The Finish Line and Post-Race Emotions

Crossing the finish line of your first marathon is an unforgettable experience, and the Chicago Marathon finish in Grant Park is particularly rewarding. The sense of accomplishment is immense, and it's common to experience a mixture of elation, relief, and pride. Allow yourself a moment to celebrate and take in the experience before heading to the post-race area for food, hydration, and recovery.

Many runners feel a "post-race high," but as adrenaline fades, fatigue will set in. Moving around and stretching gently is essential, as this helps prevent muscle stiffness. Keep warm, and drink fluids to aid in recovery.

9. Reflecting on Your Accomplishment

After the marathon, take time to reflect on the journey you've completed. Completing a marathon is a significant achievement, and it's important to acknowledge the dedication, discipline, and hard work that went into reaching the finish line. Consider keeping a journal of your experience, noting moments of personal triumph or challenge.

Many first-time marathoners report that the experience has a lasting impact, instilling a sense of confidence and resilience. Reflecting on your marathon journey can serve as a powerful motivator for future goals, whether that means setting new running targets or applying the lessons learned to other areas of life.

10. Planning for What's Next

For many runners, the first marathon is just the beginning. After a period of recovery, you may want to consider future races or even work towards completing the other races in the Abbott World Marathon Majors series. Setting a new goal, whether it's improving your time, tackling a different marathon, or trying a half-marathon, will keep your momentum going.

The Chicago Marathon will likely hold a special place in your heart as your first 26.2-mile race, and the experience will shape your future as a runner. Embrace your new identity as a marathoner, and remember that every step, from training to finish, is part of a memorable journey.

Chapter 6: *Chicago Marathon for First-Timers*

Taking on the Chicago Marathon for the first time is an experience filled with excitement, nerves, and the unknown. As a first-timer, there are countless things to consider, from understanding the course to knowing what to expect on race day. This chapter provides a comprehensive guide tailored specifically for those who are new to this race, covering every aspect from pre-race preparation to post-race celebrations, offering advice on how to make the most of this unique opportunity.

1. Understanding the Course and Environment

One of the Chicago Marathon's biggest draws is its flat and fast course, which winds through the heart of the city, showcasing iconic neighborhoods and landmarks. However, running through a bustling metropolitan area like Chicago also presents unique challenges. The weather, for instance, can vary wildly in October. Some years have seen unseasonably hot conditions, while others have welcomed runners with cooler, ideal temperatures. The winds off Lake Michigan can also affect the race; it's helpful to be prepared for changing weather and unpredictable elements.

The course itself takes runners through a mixture of urban landscapes, from skyscraper-lined streets to tree-lined avenues, creating a sense of energy that's hard to match. For a first-timer, understanding these variables and how they might impact their performance is key. Study the course map in advance and familiarize yourself with major points along the way. Know where the aid stations are located and mentally divide the race into sections, as this will make the distance feel more manageable.

2. Training Plan for First-Timers

Preparing for a marathon is a serious commitment, and first-time marathoners should allow several months to train. Many beginner training plans last about 16-20 weeks, with a gradual increase in mileage to build endurance safely. Given Chicago's flat terrain, you can focus on maintaining a steady pace rather than navigating hills. However, incorporating some speedwork and strength training will be valuable in building resilience, especially if you are aiming to hit a certain time goal.

Consistency is key, so ensure that your schedule includes long runs, which typically occur once a week. These runs not only help condition your body to handle the distance but also help you mentally adjust to spending hours on your feet. In the weeks leading up to the race, follow a "tapering" period, where you gradually decrease mileage to allow your body to recover and reach peak performance on race day.

First-timers may also consider joining a running club or finding a training group for support. Many groups in Chicago specifically cater to marathon runners and can offer a structured training plan with guidance from experienced runners and coaches. Additionally, talking to seasoned marathoners can provide valuable insight into what to expect on race day, from the starting line experience to navigating post-race recovery.

3. Choosing the Right Gear

Ensuring you have the right gear is essential. The Chicago Marathon has diverse weather conditions, so choose breathable, moisture-wicking clothing and layer as needed. For beginners, testing your gear during training is important. Marathon day is not the time to try out a new pair of shoes, shorts, or nutrition strategy, as doing so could lead to blisters or discomfort that could hinder your experience. Opt for running shoes that provide comfort and support for long distances, and ensure they are properly broken in.

Chicago's spectators are famously supportive, and the atmosphere can be highly motivating. However, this means you'll encounter noise, music, and cheering at various points along the course. Consider whether headphones will enhance your experience or if you'd rather immerse yourself fully in the environment.

4. Setting Realistic Goals

Setting achievable goals is crucial for first-timers. For some, simply finishing the marathon is an accomplishment, while others may have a specific time in mind. Whatever your goal, ensure it's realistic based on your training progress. Keep in mind that it's common for first-time marathoners to underestimate the mental and physical demands of running 26.2 miles. A helpful approach for beginners is to set a primary goal (e.g., finishing the race), a secondary goal (e.g., hitting a certain time), and an aspirational goal (e.g., setting a personal record).

While the race is known for its flat course and personal-best potential, it's best to avoid putting too much pressure on yourself. Approach the race with a mindset of celebration and achievement, rather than stress and rigid expectations.

5. Managing Pre-Race Jitters

Nervousness is natural, especially in the days leading up to your first marathon. To keep these nerves in check, stick to familiar routines and focus on logistics. Pick up your race bib and packet at the Chicago Marathon expo a day or two before race day, allowing yourself time to explore the event without rushing. This expo is also a great opportunity to connect with other first-timers and experienced marathoners, pick up last-minute gear, and get inspired by the scale and excitement of the event.

Prepare a checklist for race day, including items like your bib, timing chip, shoes, and nutrition, so you can head to the starting line feeling calm and organized. Make sure to get adequate rest in the days leading up to the race and stay hydrated.

6. The Starting Line Experience

The starting line can feel overwhelming for first-time runners, as thousands of runners gather in Grant Park to await the beginning of the race. Arriving early is essential, as there will be security checkpoints, gear check-in, and time to get settled in your designated corral. Embrace the energy around you, but remember to pace yourself. Adrenaline will be high, but it's crucial not to start too fast, which could lead to burnout later.

Take advantage of this moment to soak in the excitement. Many first-time runners report feeling a blend of anticipation and joy as they wait for the starting horn. Engage in the camaraderie around you, and keep your mental focus on the journey ahead rather than getting swept up in the fast pace of other runners.

7. Tackling Race-Day Challenges

Every marathon presents its challenges, and Chicago is no exception. First-time runners often encounter "the wall" around miles 18-22, where both physical and mental fatigue set in. Prepare for this by staying consistent with your hydration and nutrition plan, consuming fluids and energy gels or snacks at regular intervals. Knowing that this tough moment is likely to come can make it easier to push through.

Mentally, breaking down the course into manageable segments can help. Focus on reaching the next aid station, mile marker, or neighborhood, rather than thinking about the entire remaining distance. Drawing energy from the spectators and landmarks can also be a powerful motivator. For instance, seeing family and friends in the crowd or reaching a known milestone like Chinatown can help reinvigorate your spirit and keep you moving.

8. The Finish Line and Post-Race Emotions

Crossing the finish line of your first marathon is an unforgettable experience, and the Chicago Marathon finish in Grant Park is particularly rewarding. The sense of accomplishment is immense, and it's common to experience a mixture of elation, relief, and pride. Allow yourself a moment to celebrate and take in the experience before heading to the post-race area for food, hydration, and recovery.

Many runners feel a "post-race high," but as adrenaline fades, fatigue will set in. Moving around and stretching gently is essential, as this helps prevent muscle stiffness. Keep warm, and drink fluids to aid in recovery.

9. Reflecting on Your Accomplishment

After the marathon, take time to reflect on the journey you've completed. Completing a marathon is a significant achievement, and it's important to acknowledge the dedication, discipline, and hard work that went into reaching the finish line. Consider keeping a journal of your experience, noting moments of personal triumph or challenge.

Many first-time marathoners report that the experience has a lasting impact, instilling a sense of confidence and resilience. Reflecting on your marathon journey can serve as a powerful motivator for future goals, whether that means setting new running targets or applying the lessons learned to other areas of life.

10. Planning for What's Next

For many runners, the first marathon is just the beginning. After a period of recovery, you may want to consider future races or even work towards completing the other races in the Abbott World Marathon Majors series. Setting a new goal, whether it's improving your time, tackling a different marathon, or trying a half-marathon, will keep your momentum going.

The Chicago Marathon will likely hold a special place in your heart as your first 26.2-mile race, and the experience will shape your future as a runner. Embrace your new identity as a marathoner, and remember that every step, from training to finish, is part of a memorable journey.

Chapter 7: Chicago Marathon for Experienced Runners

The Chicago Marathon is a unique experience for all runners, but it holds special appeal for seasoned marathoners. Known for its flat, fast course and vibrant atmosphere, Chicago offers opportunities to chase personal bests, savor the city's rich cultural diversity, and enjoy an iconic event that's part of the Abbott World Marathon Majors. For experienced runners who are familiar with the marathon distance and have logged multiple races, this chapter explores strategies, insights, and considerations for making the most of Chicago's marathon course, refining performance goals, and enjoying the race from a seasoned perspective.

1. Setting Specific Goals for Chicago's Flat Course

With its reputation as one of the flattest courses among the major marathons, the Chicago Marathon is a favorite for runners aiming to achieve a personal record (PR) or qualify for the Boston Marathon. Experienced marathoners who have previously raced on hilly or undulating courses will find that Chicago's gentle elevation profile enables a consistent pace throughout, allowing for a focused approach toward a time goal. This relatively flat course is also more forgiving on muscles, leading to lower fatigue over time compared to races with significant climbs.

Goal-setting is a crucial part of the preparation process. Many experienced runners create specific pacing strategies for Chicago, often targeting negative splits. Starting at a controlled pace in the first half and accelerating in the latter stages can help prevent burnout and yield faster finishing times. Incorporating tempo runs and interval training into a training plan will build speed and endurance, which is advantageous for the fast-paced nature of Chicago's course.

2. Refining the Training Plan for Optimal Performance

For experienced runners, marathon training goes beyond simply completing long runs. To maximize performance on Chicago's flat course, consider a customized training plan that balances long-distance endurance with speedwork, strength training, and tapering. Given that Chicago is typically run in October, seasoned runners should plan for late-summer peak training, which may involve running in warmer conditions.

Speed sessions, such as interval training and tempo runs, are essential to prepare for the faster sections of the course. Incorporating mile repeats, 800-meter intervals, and marathon-pace runs can help you feel comfortable at a high intensity. Additionally, strength training to target core stability and lower body resilience can prevent fatigue during the latter miles. As you taper in the final weeks before race day, focus on resting, maintaining flexibility, and engaging in mental preparation.

Chicago's conditions can vary, so doing a few training runs in conditions that simulate the race environment — early mornings or cooler fall weather — will be beneficial. Additionally, training at or near marathon pace during these sessions will help your body adapt to the intensity of race day.

3. Strategic Course Navigation and Pacing

While Chicago's course is straightforward, experienced runners know that proper pacing and strategic navigation are key to optimizing performance. The Chicago Marathon course begins in Grant Park and weaves through 29 neighborhoods, making it a dynamic and engaging race that offers sights of some of the city's most iconic areas, including Lincoln Park, the Magnificent Mile, and Pilsen.

For experienced runners, the challenge lies in managing energy efficiently over the distance. Many seasoned marathoners advise against getting too caught up in the excitement of the first few miles. The enthusiastic crowd, flat terrain, and adrenaline can easily lead to an overly fast start, which can be costly in the final stages. Instead, maintain a conservative pace at the beginning, focusing on consistency and patience. By around mile 20, you'll be better positioned to pick up the pace if you have energy in reserve.

Chicago's racecourse has a few turns, especially in the downtown area, which can affect rhythm and efficiency. Practicing on courses with turns or working on foot placement can help maintain balance and control, minimizing any potential for slowing down around corners.

4. Fine-Tuning Race-Day Nutrition and Hydration

Experienced marathoners understand the importance of nutrition and hydration during long-distance races. For Chicago, preparing a well-thought-out plan that aligns with the race's aid stations is essential. Aid stations are located approximately every 1-2 miles along the course, stocked with water and sports drinks. Knowing the locations of these stations ahead of time can help you plan when and where to hydrate.

Experienced runners often carry their preferred gels or energy supplements, using the aid stations for hydration. Start hydrating early in the race to maintain electrolyte balance and avoid energy crashes. Test various gels, chews, or other nutritional options during training to determine what works best for your body and won't upset your stomach on race day.

For many runners, Chicago's cooler October weather can be an advantage, reducing the risk of dehydration compared to summer marathons. However, because Chicago's temperatures can fluctuate, it's best to adapt your hydration based on the weather forecast leading up to race day.

5. Leveraging Chicago's Crowd Support and Energy

The Chicago Marathon's vibrant atmosphere is powered by thousands of spectators who line the course, cheering runners on from start to finish. Experienced marathoners often describe the energy in Chicago as an advantage, giving them a mental boost when needed most. As you move through neighborhoods like Boystown, where the cheers are particularly lively, use the crowd's energy as motivation to keep your pace strong.

For seasoned runners, interacting with the crowd can be a strategic way to manage energy levels. In quieter sections, focus inwardly on pacing and form. When the crowd intensifies in areas like Chinatown and near the finish line in Grant Park, let the energy fuel you to push through any fatigue. The enthusiastic support, especially during the challenging final miles, is invaluable.

6. Planning Logistics for Maximum Efficiency

Experienced runners know that logistics play a significant role in marathon success. Plan your pre-race routine carefully, from transportation to gear preparation. Arrive at the starting line early enough to allow time for security checks, gear drop-off, and a proper warm-up. Knowing the layout of Grant Park, where the race begins and ends, will streamline your morning.

Additionally, consider your post-race logistics. Chicago's finish line area can be crowded, and organizing a meeting point with family or friends can help avoid stress after the race. Preparing for post-race refueling and recovery, such as keeping a jacket or nutrition at the gear check, ensures you can quickly begin recovering after crossing the finish line.

7. Mastering the Mental Side of Marathon Racing

Seasoned marathoners know that success in the marathon is as much mental as it is physical. The Chicago Marathon offers an ideal environment for mental resilience, thanks to its supportive crowd and scenic course. Yet, as every runner knows, the final miles of a marathon present mental challenges that can make or break a race.

Visualization techniques are popular among experienced runners. By visualizing the course and imagining key moments, such as crossing the finish line, you can mentally prepare for the emotions you'll experience. Also, create a mantra or mental cue to use when you encounter tough moments. Focus on reaching the next mile marker or aid station, breaking the race into smaller, manageable parts.

Another approach is to use the scenery as a mental reset. For instance, when reaching an iconic area like the Magnificent Mile, take a moment to appreciate the atmosphere. The ability to stay present can make the race feel shorter and keep your spirits high.

8. Celebrating Achievements and Reflecting on the Experience

For experienced runners, crossing the finish line at the Chicago Marathon is a moment of pride. The achievement isn't just about completing 26.2 miles but also about the months of preparation, the disciplined training, and the ability to overcome the physical and mental challenges of race day. Reflect on your goals and whether you met or exceeded your expectations.

Chicago is known for its post-race festivities, including celebrations within Grant Park and surrounding neighborhoods. Many experienced runners celebrate their finish by reconnecting with fellow runners or indulging in a post-race meal. Take time to savor the accomplishment, whether you hit a PR or simply enjoyed the race from start to finish.

9. Analyzing Performance and Setting Future Goals

After the race, experienced runners typically conduct a performance analysis to identify strengths and areas for improvement. Reviewing data from GPS watches, pace charts, and race splits can help determine where energy was well-spent and where adjustments could be made. Reflecting on nutrition, hydration, and pacing strategies provides insights to fine-tune for future races.

Some experienced runners may use Chicago as a benchmark for other marathons or for setting future goals. Whether it's achieving an even faster time or applying lessons learned to more challenging races, reviewing your performance after Chicago is a valuable exercise. Many seasoned marathoners take this time to consider additional Abbott World Marathon Majors races or challenging terrains to keep their marathon journey fresh and fulfilling.

10. Chicago as Part of a Marathoner's Journey

For seasoned runners, the Chicago Marathon is often more than a single race; it becomes part of a lifelong journey in the sport. Completing this marathon not only builds one's credentials within the running community but also provides memories that last a lifetime. Whether you aim to complete all six major marathons or simply enjoy Chicago's unique energy, every runner takes something meaningful away from this experience.

Each time you return to Chicago, you bring a new level of experience and insight, making each marathon a unique encounter. Embrace the journey as a testament to your dedication and passion for the sport, and let the city's incredible support fuel future ambitions in your marathon journey.

Chapter 8: Chicago Marathon's Role in the Major Six

The Abbott World Marathon Majors is a prestigious series that includes six of the most iconic marathons in the world: Boston, London, Berlin, Chicago, New York City, and Tokyo. Known collectively as the "Big Six," these races bring together elite athletes and passionate runners alike, creating some of the most competitive and celebrated events in marathon history. Among these, the Chicago Marathon holds a unique place due to its history, the nature of its course, and the level of participation it attracts. For runners striving to complete all six races, Chicago serves as a crucial experience that stands out in both its accessibility and reputation as a personal best (PB) course.

This chapter explores how the Chicago Marathon fits into the global framework of the Major Six, examining its distinct characteristics, its appeal to various types of runners, and its role in the journey of runners pursuing the Major Six stars. By understanding Chicago's role in this elite series, runners can better appreciate its importance and prepare for what is often one of the most memorable marathons in their careers.

1. An Essential Race in the Majors Lineup

The Chicago Marathon has been part of the Abbott World Marathon Majors since the series was launched in 2006, and it has remained a pillar of the series ever since. For runners aiming to earn the Six Star Medal — awarded to those who complete all six Major Marathons — Chicago is often seen as one of the most approachable races. Unlike Boston, which requires qualifying times, or Tokyo, which has limited international entries, Chicago is accessible through a lottery system, charity spots, and even guaranteed entries for those with qualifying times. This accessibility has cemented Chicago's role as a key race in achieving the Six Star Medal, allowing a diverse range of runners to participate.

Chicago's prominence in the Majors lineup has also helped elevate its reputation globally. Runners from over 100 countries participate each year, contributing to the international atmosphere that sets the race apart. The diversity of participants makes Chicago a melting pot of cultures, bringing together runners who share a common goal: to compete in one of the best marathon courses in the world as part of the Major Six challenge.

2. The Chicago Course: A Flat and Fast Route Ideal for PBs

The Chicago Marathon's course is renowned for being one of the flattest in the Major Six series, making it an ideal race for runners aiming to achieve personal records or qualifying times for other races, such as Boston. Starting and ending in Grant Park, the route takes runners through 29 neighborhoods, showcasing both Chicago's urban and scenic appeal without major changes in elevation. This allows runners to maintain a steady pace and encourages record-breaking performances.

Many elite runners and record chasers turn to Chicago for its reputation as a "fast course." In 2019, Brigid Kosgei of Kenya set a new women's marathon world record here, breaking a 16-year standing record. For elite athletes, Chicago's flat course, combined with the high energy of cheering crowds, creates the ideal conditions to push the limits of what's possible. Likewise, for amateur runners, it offers an opportunity to test their potential and set goals within a structured and supportive environment.

In comparison, courses in New York and Boston present unique challenges with their hills and bridges, while London and Berlin offer other appeals, such as scenic historic landmarks and similarly fast conditions. Still, Chicago's distinction lies in the balance it strikes between accessibility, crowd support, and ideal conditions for fast times.

3. Crowd Support and Cultural Richness of Chicago

One of the standout aspects of the Chicago Marathon is the enthusiastic crowd support, a feature shared by many of the Majors but particularly emphasized in Chicago. The race route's design takes runners through a vibrant mix of neighborhoods, each offering a unique flavor and style of support. From the energy of Boystown to the rhythms of Pilsen, the crowd experience is a highlight of the Chicago Marathon, making it memorable for both experienced marathoners and first-timers.

The cultural diversity of Chicago is on full display during race day. Spectators from diverse backgrounds bring a unique energy to the course, creating a festive atmosphere that keeps runners motivated. Whether it's the drumbeats, traditional dance troupes, or cheering residents, the supportive crowd provides a level of encouragement that resonates with runners and keeps them pushing forward. For runners who have already completed other Major Marathons, this aspect of Chicago sets it apart as a warm and welcoming course.

This vibrant atmosphere is echoed in New York and London, but Chicago's layout through various ethnic neighborhoods — from Chinatown to Little Italy — offers a unique, inclusive representation of the city's spirit. Experienced marathoners frequently note that Chicago's crowd support is one of the best in the series, and this energy makes it a distinct experience within the Major Six.

4. Chicago's Influence on Marathon Accessibility and Charity Participation

The Chicago Marathon's accessibility extends beyond its flat course. Unlike other Majors that require rigorous qualification, Chicago embraces a wider spectrum of runners, including a robust charity program that enables participants to secure entries while supporting causes they care about. This charity model has inspired similar approaches in other Majors, such as London and New York, promoting marathon participation as a philanthropic opportunity.

Chicago's charity program has made the marathon more inclusive, allowing individuals who might not meet qualifying times to participate while raising significant funds for charitable organizations. Each year, Chicago's charity runners contribute millions of dollars, making a substantial impact in areas such as health research, community development, and global humanitarian causes. For runners striving to complete the Major Six, Chicago offers a gateway to both personal achievement and meaningful impact.

Compared to other Majors, Chicago's charity program is one of the most developed, offering numerous options for entry and extensive support for participants. This inclusiveness has contributed to Chicago's appeal within the Major Six, attracting both seasoned marathoners and philanthropic runners alike.

5. The Role of the Chicago Marathon in Marathon History

The Chicago Marathon holds a significant place in marathon history, not only as a part of the Major Six but also as a pioneering event in terms of inclusivity and athletic achievement. Since its establishment in 1977, Chicago has grown from a local race into an internationally acclaimed event. Its consistent commitment to quality and support for world-class performances has made it a staple of the marathon world, drawing elites and amateurs alike.

The Chicago Marathon's role in breaking records has cemented its reputation as a top-tier marathon. Over the years, athletes like Khalid Khannouchi and Brigid Kosgei have made history in Chicago, raising the event's profile and setting it apart within the Majors. This legacy of excellence continues to attract competitive runners, reinforcing Chicago's importance within the Major Six series.

6. Comparing Chicago with the Other Major Marathons

Each of the six Major Marathons offers something unique, and Chicago's defining features make it a compelling choice for runners seeking specific goals. Boston's hills, Berlin's consistent record-breaking potential, and New York's intense crowd support all have their appeals, but Chicago's flat course and diverse neighborhoods create a special atmosphere.

Experienced runners who have completed other Majors often cite Chicago as one of the best races for a PB attempt, while Berlin's flat course is similar but often more crowded due to limited entry slots. Boston and Tokyo present greater challenges for entry, and their race-day conditions can vary drastically, whereas Chicago tends to provide consistent, mild October weather conducive to fast times.

7. Chicago's Impact on a Runner's Major Six Journey

For those aiming to achieve the coveted Six Star Medal, Chicago often represents a key step along the journey. Its accessibility and inclusive approach make it one of the first Major Marathons many runners tackle. Successfully completing Chicago can boost a runner's confidence, providing them with experience in a large-scale race and setting a foundation for tackling more challenging races like Boston or New York.

The Chicago Marathon is often an early stepping stone for runners who go on to complete all six Majors. Its welcoming nature and focus on personal bests allow runners to develop essential marathon skills while joining a larger community of runners who share similar ambitions.

8. The Economic and Cultural Impact of Chicago as a Major Marathon

The Chicago Marathon's influence extends beyond the running community. Each year, the event contributes significantly to the local economy, drawing international visitors, bolstering tourism, and engaging local businesses. From hotels to restaurants, Chicago's economy benefits substantially, showcasing how the race has a lasting impact on the city itself.

The marathon also brings communities together, fostering a sense of local pride and civic engagement. As residents cheer on participants from all over the world, the race serves as a reminder of Chicago's inclusivity and resilience, characteristics that distinguish it within the Major Six.

9. The Significance of Earning the Six Star Medal at Chicago

For runners striving to complete all Major Marathons, crossing the finish line at Chicago is often a monumental achievement. Chicago is a gateway to the Six Star journey, providing a positive race-day experience and the resources needed to succeed in larger, more challenging marathons. Completing Chicago gives runners a sense of accomplishment that propels them toward the other races in the series.

10. Chicago's Legacy in the World of Marathon Running

The Chicago Marathon continues to play an essential role in the marathon world. Its accessibility, fast course, and supportive crowd make it a race beloved by beginners and elites alike. As part of the Major Six, Chicago is integral to the sport, exemplifying the potential of large-scale marathon events and inspiring runners to push their limits. Whether as a first step in the Six Star journey or a personal best destination, Chicago's legacy endures, offering a premier marathon experience that draws runners back year after year.

Conclusion: The Chicago Marathon's Enduring Legacy

The Bank of America Chicago Marathon stands as one of the most celebrated events in the global marathon circuit, with a legacy that transcends generations and continues to grow. Through its unique combination of accessibility, inclusivity, and competitive spirit, the Chicago Marathon has established itself as a race that appeals to runners of all backgrounds and abilities, from seasoned elites chasing world records to first-time marathoners eager to experience the thrill of a world-class event. With its reputation as a flat, fast course that traverses one of America's most vibrant cities, it's no wonder that the Chicago Marathon has become a must-do for marathoners worldwide.

This iconic race is not just a sporting event but also a cultural celebration that showcases the diversity, resilience, and charm of Chicago itself. The marathon brings together individuals from all walks of life, creating an atmosphere of camaraderie and shared passion for the sport. Spectators lining the course and cheering runners through 29 unique neighborhoods are an integral part of what makes the Chicago Marathon experience unforgettable. In this conclusion, we reflect on the many elements that contribute to Chicago's enduring legacy and its significance in the world of long-distance running, especially as a member of the esteemed Abbott World Marathon Majors.

1. A Race for Everyone: Inclusivity and Accessibility

The Chicago Marathon is often celebrated as one of the most accessible events among the Major Six. Unlike the Boston Marathon, which requires a stringent qualifying time, or the Tokyo Marathon, with its limited international entries, Chicago offers a lottery system, time-based entry options, and charity slots. This range of entry methods allows runners of all skill levels to participate, making the race accessible to individuals who might not otherwise have the chance to run in a world-class marathon. Charity participation, in particular, has expanded the race's reach, enabling runners to support causes they believe in while taking part in an iconic event.

This inclusivity resonates with runners around the world, making the Chicago Marathon a race that attracts participants from more than 100 countries each year. By giving individuals the chance to participate in a major race without the daunting challenge of qualifying times, Chicago has opened the door for many runners who seek to test their limits in a marathon setting. This openness also reinforces the marathon's place as a welcoming event, where personal accomplishment and community support stand as key pillars.

2. Chicago's Unmatched Course for Personal Bests

The Chicago Marathon has gained a reputation as one of the best races in the world for setting a personal best, thanks to its flat course, favorable October weather, and minimal elevation changes. Many runners target the Chicago Marathon with the hope of achieving their fastest times. Whether it's elite athletes pushing for world records or amateur runners aiming for personal bests, Chicago provides a course conducive to peak performance. The city's streets allow runners to establish a rhythm and maintain a steady pace, while the enthusiastic crowd support further boosts performance.

Runners looking to qualify for the Boston Marathon often turn to Chicago as a race to meet their goal. With each passing year, Chicago solidifies its place in the marathon world as a personal best destination, fostering a competitive atmosphere that drives runners to perform at their highest level. This focus on personal achievement has become a hallmark of the Chicago Marathon, aligning with the race's broader mission of making marathon running a rewarding and accessible pursuit for all.

3. The Importance of the Chicago Marathon in the Major Six Journey

As part of the Abbott World Marathon Majors, the Chicago Marathon plays a pivotal role in the journey of runners aiming to complete all six major marathons. For those who aspire to earn the Six Star Medal, Chicago is often one of the first milestones due to its accessibility and reputation as a well-organized, runner-friendly event. The city's race attracts thousands of marathoners each year who are committed to this ambitious goal, contributing to the marathon's reputation as a key stepping stone in the Major Six journey.

Completing the Chicago Marathon instills confidence in runners as they prepare for the unique challenges posed by the other Major Marathons. Chicago serves as an ideal proving ground where runners can gain experience in a large-scale, high-energy marathon while also working toward a greater objective. The race's seamless organization, robust support, and engaged spectators offer a supportive environment that inspires runners to tackle the remaining marathons in the series with renewed motivation and drive.

4. Economic and Cultural Impact on the City of Chicago

The economic impact of the Chicago Marathon on the city is substantial, generating millions of dollars in revenue each year from tourism, hospitality, and local spending. The influx of international visitors boosts hotel bookings, restaurant reservations, and spending at local businesses, benefiting the city's economy and providing an annual highlight for many Chicago establishments. This financial impact extends to the broader community, as the marathon creates jobs, supports local vendors, and brings an influx of energy and excitement to the city each October.

Culturally, the marathon is more than just a race; it's an event that embodies the spirit of Chicago, showcasing the city's pride, unity, and inclusivity. Each neighborhood on the course brings its unique identity to the event, offering runners a glimpse into the city's diverse communities. The marathon has become a point of pride for Chicagoans, who turn out in droves to support the runners, whether they are locals or international participants. This community support and cultural representation make the Chicago Marathon a uniquely enriching experience, reflecting the essence of the city itself.

5. A Legacy of Record-Breaking Performances and World-Class Competition

Chicago's history of record-breaking performances has elevated it to the status of a competitive marathon on par with Berlin, Tokyo, and New York. The marathon has witnessed numerous world records and personal achievements, with elite athletes often choosing Chicago to make their mark. In 2019, Brigid Kosgei's world record for the women's marathon solidified Chicago's reputation as a fast, competitive course that attracts top talent from around the globe. This competitive atmosphere has drawn elite runners seeking optimal conditions and motivated amateur runners who want to challenge themselves alongside the best.

The marathon's competitive legacy inspires runners of all levels to push their limits. Knowing they're running in the footsteps of record-holders and world-class athletes gives participants a unique sense of connection to the sport's history and accomplishments. Chicago's role in advancing the field of competitive marathon running has positioned it as a leading event that continues to shape the future of the sport.

6. Looking Ahead: The Future of the Chicago Marathon

As the marathon world evolves, the Chicago Marathon remains a leader in innovation, accessibility, and inclusivity. The event organizers continue to prioritize runner experience, ensuring that each year's race is more seamless, supportive, and enjoyable than the last. With ongoing efforts to improve sustainability, embrace technological advancements, and enhance crowd engagement, the Chicago Marathon is well-positioned to continue its legacy for future generations of runners.

The marathon's commitment to excellence and inclusivity means that it will remain a key destination for runners from around the world, helping them achieve their goals and celebrate their love for the sport. In a world where marathon running is increasingly popular, the Chicago Marathon stands as an event that adapts to meet the needs of its diverse participant base, setting a benchmark for other races to follow.

7. The Chicago Marathon's Lasting Legacy

The Chicago Marathon's place in the Major Six and its role as a personal best destination, a cultural celebration, and a champion of inclusivity all contribute to its lasting legacy. For many runners, completing the Chicago Marathon is more than a personal achievement; it's a lifelong memory shaped by the support of spectators, the thrill of the course, and the pride of finishing a world-class event. This marathon leaves a lasting impact on everyone who participates, motivating runners to return year after year and inspiring future generations to embrace the joy of long-distance running.

As one of the world's most iconic races, the Chicago Marathon symbolizes the enduring appeal of marathon running, uniting people from diverse backgrounds in the pursuit of a common goal. Whether it's a first marathon or a journey toward the Six Star Medal, the Chicago Marathon offers an unparalleled experience that runners carry with them, strengthening their connection to the sport and the city of Chicago. The marathon's legacy is built on the achievements of its participants, the dedication of its organizers, and the spirit of the community that supports it — a legacy that will endure for years to come.

Printed in Dunstable, United Kingdom